Basic Study Designs in Epidemiology: Concept Maps to Stimulate Learning

D. Faulkner PhD MPH

ISBN: 1479369551
ISBN 13: 9781479369553
Library of Congress Control Number: 2012917850
CreateSpace, North Charleston, SC

Table of Contents

Introduction

Epidemiology is the study of the distribution and determinants of health-related events in human populations and the application of this study to control health problems. In order to conduct research in this field, the investigator first specifies a question that he or she wants to answer, such as "Does cigarette smoking lead to lung cancer?" The research question represents the investigator's idea of how nature works.

In order for this research question to be answered, however, it must be translated into testable, measurable observations. The analytic study design is the vehicle for that translation; it is the equivalent of a recipe or blueprint of a building.

This book is a student's guide to basic analytic study designs. It is meant to serve as a supplemental resource for those who are taking formal courses in disciplines such as epidemiology, health statistics, and demography. It can also serve as an on-the-job reference manual for practitioners.

To enhance understanding, I have structured information in the forms of outlines, definitions, tables, formulas, and quizzes. The most powerful information structure is the concept map, which is a diagram illustrating how terms and ideas interconnect. I find concept maps to be very powerful learning tools, and I trust that you will agree after using this handbook.

"Practice, the master of all things"
—Augustus Octavius

—D. Faulkner

Lesson 1: Scales of Measurement

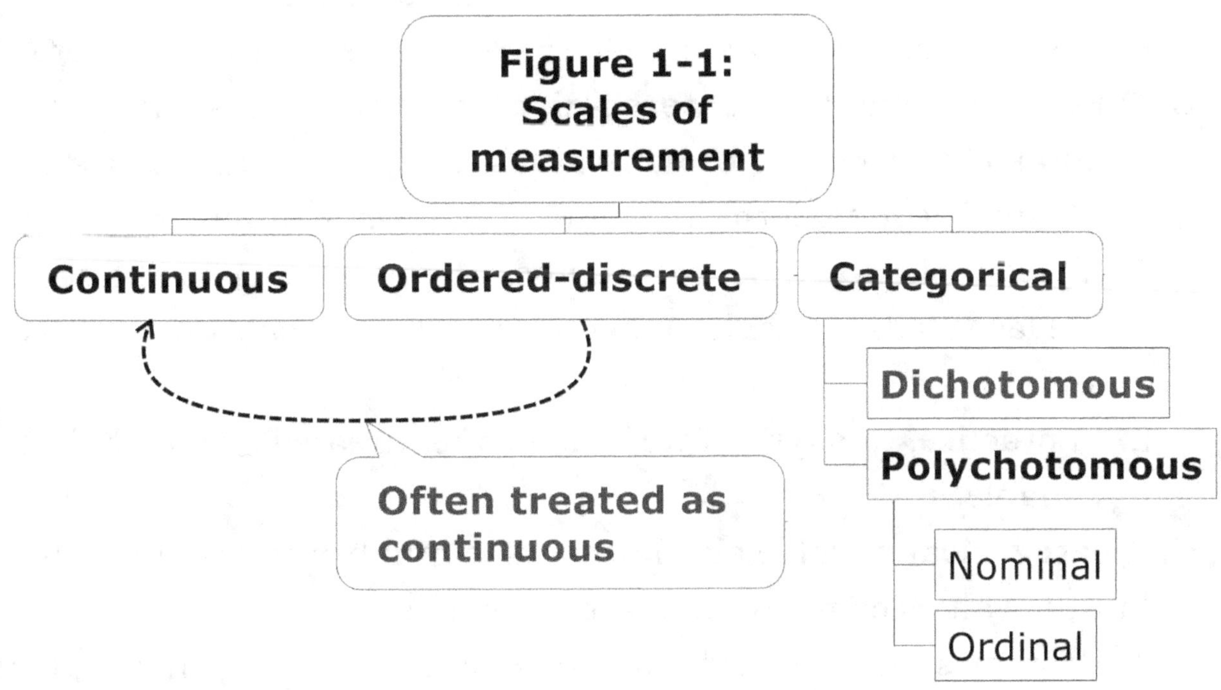

1) Summary

- Variables are the building blocks of research.
- This lesson introduces the concept of a variable and describes how variables are structured.

2) What is a variable?

- A **variable** is an attribute that differentiates members of a group or set.
- This attribute takes on different values.
- For instance, age, gender, and ethnicity are variables.

3) How are variables structured?

I. There are three broad structures or measurement scales: continuous, ordered-discrete, and categorical (Figure 1-1).

A. A **continuous** variable has an infinite (or countless) number of possible values along a continuum, and the values can be in fractional form.

1. An example would be "weight in pounds," which could have values such as 100, 100.5, 154, 154.9, 159, 209, 432, et cetera.

B. On the other hand, an **ordered-discrete** variable has a finite (or countable) number of possible values. In addition, the values cannot be in fractional form; they must be in whole numbers.

1. An example would be "the number of days one smoked during the last 30 days," which could have values such as 0, 1, 2, 10, and 30.
2. In practice, this type of variable is often treated as a continuous variable.

C. A **categorical** variable also has a finite number of possible values, but the values come from preset categories.

1. Examples include gender (male, female) and yearly income (low, medium, high).
2. Categorical variables with two possible values are termed **dichotomous**.
3. Categorical variables with more than two possible values are termed **polychotomous**.

a) Gender (male, female) is an example of a dichotomous variable, while yearly income (low, medium, high) is an example of a polychotomous variable.

b) Polychotomous variables can be further characterized by the nature of the categories (Figure 1-1).

II. **Nominal** variables have no particular order of importance among the categories.

A. An example of this type of variable is the region of the country (North, South, East, West).

III. With **ordinal** variables, there is an implied rank-order among the categories.

A. An example of this type of variable is the degree of pain (severe, moderate, mild).

B. One commonly used ordinal measure is the **Likert scale**, which asks individuals to describe their attitudes about an object, event, issue, or person.

1. An example of a Likert scale item would be: "Smoking cigarettes is dangerous to one's health" (strongly agree, agree, neither agree nor disagree, disagree, strongly disagree).

4) What are the features of a well-designed categorical variable?

I. The categories that are present should be exhaustive and mutually exclusive.

A. If the categories are **exhaustive**, then there is a category to hold every possible observation.

1. A nonexhaustive example is the variable "body weight" (over-weight, about the right weight).

a) The category for "underweight" is missing.

b) Thus, this variable is not exhaustive.

B. If the categories are **mutually exclusive**, then no observation can be logically placed in more than one category.
   1. A non-mutually-exclusive example is the variable "age in years" using the categories 18–39, 39–59, 60–89, 90 or more.
      a) People who are 39 years of age could fit into the first category and the second category.
      b) Therefore, these categories are not mutually exclusive.
      c) To fix the variable, the categories could be 18–39, 40–59, 60–89, and 90 or more.

5) Which measurement scale is the most informative?

I. The continuous (or ordered-discrete) structure contains the most information and the dichotomous structure has the least (Figure 1-1).

II. Polychotomous variables offer an intermediate level of **informativeness**, with ordinal variables offering more information than nominal variables.

III. For instance, say that an investigator wants to compare the effects of Treatment A versus Treatment B on systolic blood pressure (SBP) across study subjects.
   A. Measuring SBP in millimeters of mercury (continuous scale) during the data collection phase would better allow the investigator to estimate treatment effects on SBP at the data analysis phase.
   B. On the other hand, measuring SBP on a dichotomous scale (low or normal versus high) during the data collection phase would limit the investigator's ability to estimate treatment effects on SBP at the data analysis phase.

Quiz 1

Questions 1–7

For each numbered variable below, identify the ONE best lettered response. Each letter may be used once, more than once, or not at all.

A. Polychotomous-nominal
B. Polychotomous-ordinal
C. Dichotomous
D. Continuous
E. Ordered-discrete

1. Place of residence (North, South, East, West):
2. Likert scale representing your comfort working with a person who has AIDS (strongly agree, agree, no opinion, disagree, strongly disagree):
3. Height in inches:
4. Sex (male, female):
5. Weight in pounds:
6. Age (0–10, 11–20, 21–30 years):
7. Age in years:

8. Which statement below properly ranks the scales of measurement from the highest to the lowest level of informativeness?

   A. Dichotomous, polychotomous, continuous
   B. Continuous, polychotomous, dichotomous
   C. Polychotomous, dichotomous, continuous
   D. Polychotomous, continuous, dichotomous

9. It is usually best to use the highest level of informativeness possible for each variable.

   A. True
   B. False

Questions 10–14
Consider a survey measuring the age of a child:

10. What is the scale of measurement of Survey Item 1?

    A. Polychotomous
    B. Dichotomous
    C. Continuous

> **Survey Item 1**
> "Which age group best represents the age (in years) of the patient?"
>
> a. 0-3
> b. 4-11
> c. 12-17
>
> **Survey Item 2**
> "What is the age of the patient in years?" ____

11. What is the scale of measurement of Survey Item 2?

    A. Polychotomous
    B. Dichotomous
    C. Continuous

12. Which survey item is the more desirable in terms of informativeness?

    A. Survey Item 1
    B. Survey Item 2

13. The response options for Survey Item 1 are:

    A. Mutually exclusive
    B. Exhaustive
    C. Mutually exclusive and exhaustive
    D. Not applicable, because "age" isn't a categorical variable here

14. The response options for Survey Item 2 are:

    A. Mutually exclusive
    B. Exhaustive
    C. Mutually exclusive and exhaustive
    D. Not applicable because "age" isn't a categorical variable here

Quiz 1–Answers

1. A
2. B
3. D
4. C
5. D
6. B; people can be ranked by "degree of" age
7. D
8. B
9. A
10. A
11. C
12. B
13. C
14. D

Lesson 2: From Variables to Research Questions

1) Summary

- In Lesson 1, you were introduced to "variables" and how they are structured.
- In Lesson 2, you will learn that variables are the building blocks of the research question.

2) What is a research question?

I. A **research question** is the question that the investigator wants to answer by doing the project.

A. There are two broad types of research questions: descriptive and analytic (or etiologic).

1. **Descriptive** research questions aim to profile the magnitude and characteristics of a phenomenon. More specifically, they aim to describe phenomena with respect to "magnitude," "person," "place," and "time."

a) Examples of such research questions include:

(1) What is the prevalence of teenage distracted driving in the United States? (magnitude)

(2) How does the prevalence of teenage distracted driving differ by gender? (person)

(3) How does teenage distracted driving occurrence vary by geographic location? (place)

(4) How has the prevalence of teenage distracted driving changed from year to year? (time)

b) Descriptive research questions provide an understanding of the *baseline* situation.

2. Analytic (or etiologic) research questions are extensions of descriptive research questions.

a) The investigator goes beyond describing the phenomenon to striving to identify specific risk factors for or protective factors against the phenomenon (health condition).

b) An example of an analytic research question is "Among teenagers, are smokers more likely to engage in distracted driving behavior than non-smokers?" In this question, smoking is believed to be a risk factor for distracted driving among teenagers.

3) What are the four required ingredients of an analytic research question?

I. There are four required ingredients in an analytic research question: the independent variable, the dependent variable, the target population, and the conceptual hypothesis (Figure 2-1).

A. The **independent variable** is the factor that *influences* an event. Synonyms include "**exposure variable**" and "**predictor variable.**"

B. The **dependent variable** is the event that is influenced. Synonyms include "**disease variable,**" "**outcome variable,**" and "**response variable.**"

C. The **target population** refers to the group of individuals to which the study results apply.

1. Recall the previous example of an analytic research question: "Among teenagers, are smokers more likely to engage in distracted driving behavior than non-smokers?"
   a) Here, the independent variable is "smoking."
   b) The dependent variable is "distracted driving."
   c) The target population is "teenagers."

D. A **conceptual hypothesis** is a tentative answer to the research question that is specified before the study begins.

1. Note that ultimately a hypothesis may or may not be supported by the study's findings.
2. Hypotheses have three possible directions of association: positive, negative, and null.
   a) The hypothesis indicates a **positive association** when it suggests that the dependent variable increases as the independent variable increases, or that the dependent variable decreases as the independent variable decreases.
      (1) An example would be this hypothesis: "As years of smoking increase, the risk of developing lung cancer will increase."
   b) The hypothesis indicates a **negative (or inverse) association** if it suggests that the dependent variable decreases as the independent variable increases, or that the dependent variable increases as the independent variable decreases.
      (1) An example would be this hypothesis: "Teen smoking will decrease as years of parental education increase."
   c) The hypothesis indicates a **null association** when it suggests that there is no relationship between the independent and dependent variables.

(1) An example would be this hypothesis: "Knowledge about the health effects of smoking will have no effect on smoking behavior."

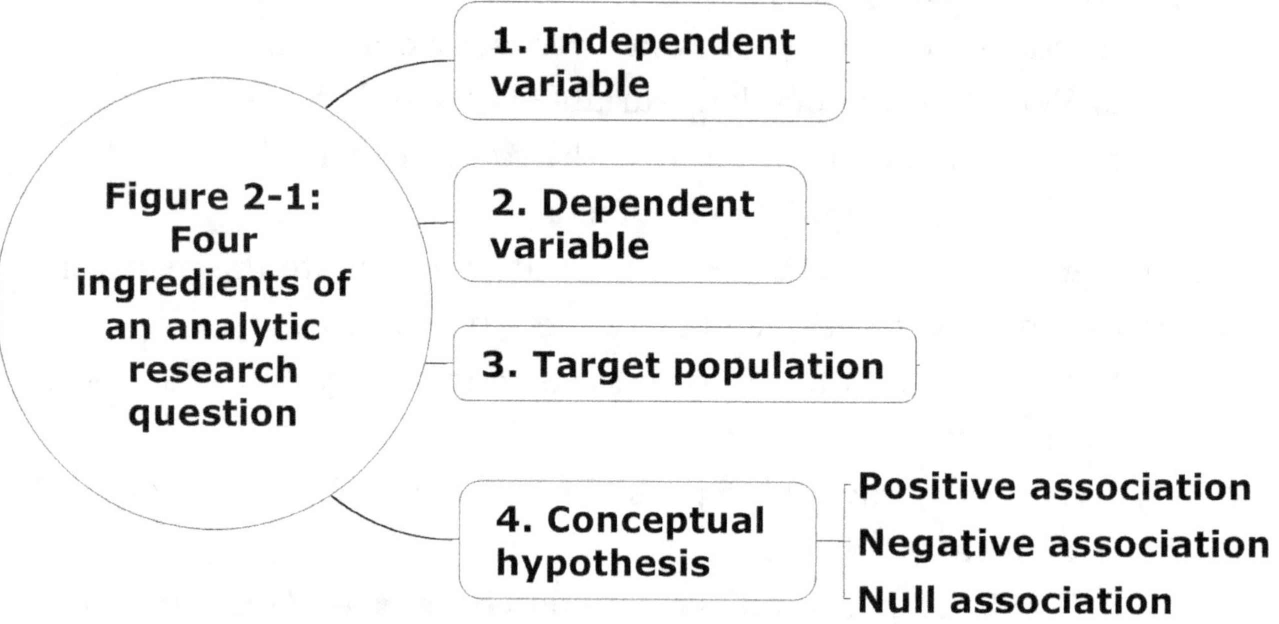

Quiz 2

Questions 1–3
Investigators hypothesize that among African-Americans, as the level of literacy increases, physical health increases.

1. What is the exposure variable?

    A. Literacy
    B. Physical health
    C. Race/ethnicity
    D. Investigators

2. What is the disease variable?

    A. Literacy
    B. Physical health
    C. Race/ethnicity
    D. Investigators

3. What is the hypothesized direction of association?

    A. Positive
    B. Negative
    C. Null

Questions 4–6
Investigators hypothesize that the more yoga one does, the lower the risk of developing osteoporosis, despite one's economic status.

4. What is the exposure variable?

    A. Economic status
    B. Yoga
    C. Osteoporosis
    D. Investigators

5. What is the disease variable?

A. Economic status
B. Yoga
C. Osteoporosis
D. Investigators

6. What is the hypothesized direction of association?

A. Positive
B. Negative
C. Null

Quiz 2–Answers

1. A
2. B
3. A
4. B
5. C
6. B

Lesson 3: Analytic Study Designs and the 2-by-2 Table

1) Summary

- In Lesson 1, you were introduced to "variables" and how they are structured.
- In Lesson 2, you learned that variables are the building blocks of the research question (descriptive versus analytic/etiologic).
- Here, we will focus on analytic research questions and discuss how they are operationalized by a countable number of analytic study designs (or "blueprints"). The standard 2-by-2 table is the unifying framework of all of the blueprints.

2) Lesson 2 describes the analytic (or etiologic) research question. Given such a question, how do we go about getting it answered?

I. The conceptual hypothesis specified in the analytic research question represents our *idea* of how nature works.

A. We must then translate that idea into testable, measurable observations.

1. The **analytic study design** is the vehicle for that translation.
   a) It bridges the gap between "thinking" and "doing" (Figure 3-1).
   b) It is the equivalent of a blueprint of a house, a roadmap, or recipe.

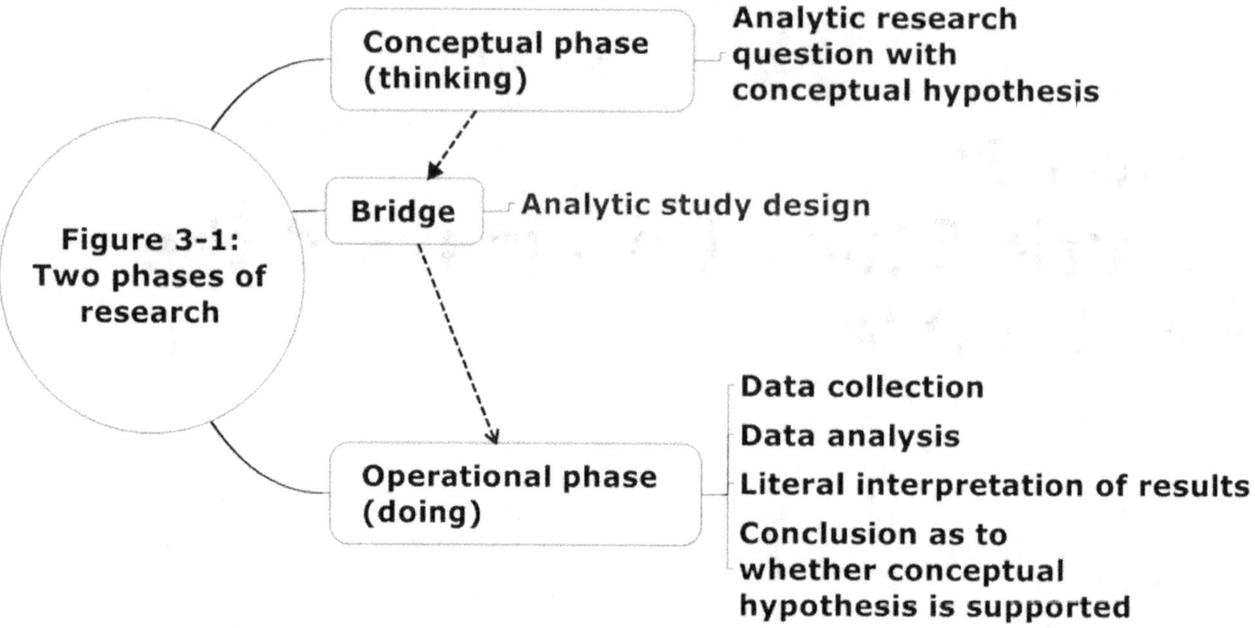

3) How many different study designs are there to choose from?

I. There are three basic study designs: the cross-sectional design, the population-based prospective cohort design, and the population-based case-control design.

A. There are also two design variations, called the retrospective cohort design and the hospital-based case-control design (Figure 3-2).

II. Lessons 4–6 will describe each study design in more detail.

III. However, before we do that, it is necessary to introduce a framework that unifies all of the study designs. It is called the standard 2-by-2 table.

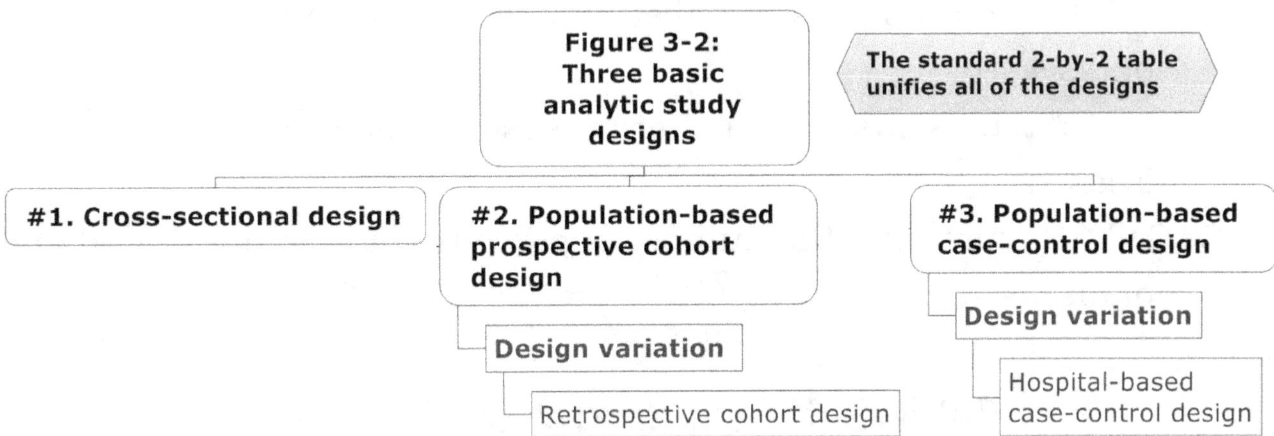

4) What is a standard 2-by-2 table?

I. The **standard 2-by-2 table** is a tabular, cross-classification of data used when both the exposure and disease variables are dichotomous (Table 3-1). Note that the columns represent disease status (yes, no) and that the rows represent exposure status (yes, no). The "~" means "not."

II. Two of the cells are called the **row marginal totals**.

A. The total number exposed is represented by a + b.

B. The total number unexposed is represented by c + d.

III. Two other cells are called the **column marginal totals**.

A. The total number of individuals with disease is represented by a + c.

B. The total number without disease is represented by b + d.

IV. Cell "n" represents the **grand total** number of individuals in the study.

V. The cells within the table represent the cross-classification of exposure and disease.

A. Thus, cell "a" represents the number of persons who are exposed and diseased.

B. Cell "b" represents the number of persons who are exposed and nondiseased.

C. Cell "c" represents the number of persons who are unexposed and diseased.

D. Cell "d" represents the number of persons who are unexposed and nondiseased.

Table 3-1: Standard 2-by-2 table

	Diseased (D, or D=1)	Nondiseased (D~, or D=0)	Total
Exposed (E, or E=1)	a	b	a + b Row 1 marginal total
Unexposed (E~, or E=0)	c	d	c + d Row 2 marginal total
Total	a + c Column 1 marginal total	b + d Column 2 marginal total	n = a + b + c + d Grand total

5) Which proportions (or percentages) can be calculated from a 2-by-2 table?

- See Tables 3-2A through 3-2D.

Table 3-2A: Joint probabilities generated from the standard 2-by-2 table

Joint probabilities	Probability notation	Cell formula
Proportion exposed and diseased	P (E and D)	a/n
Proportion exposed and nondiseased	P (E and D~)	b/n
Proportion unexposed and diseased	P (E~ and D)	c/n
Proportion unexposed and nondiseased	P (E~ and D~)	d/n

Table 3-2B: Marginal probabilities generated from the standard 2-by-2 table

Marginal probabilities	Probability notation	Cell formula
Proportion exposed	P (E)	(a + b) /n
Proportion unexposed	P (E~)	(c + d) /n
Proportion diseased	P (D)	(a + c) /n
Proportion nondiseased	P (D~)	(b + d) /n

Table 3-2C: Probabilities conditional on exposure status generated from the standard 2-by-2 table

Conditional probabilities	Probability notation	Cell formula
Proportion diseased, given exposure	P (D/E)	a/(a + b)
Proportion nondiseased, given exposure	P (D~/E)	b/(a + b)
Proportion diseased, given nonexposure	P (D/E~)	c/(c + d)
Proportion nondiseased, given nonexposure	P (D~/E~)	d/(c + d)

Table 3-2D: Probabilities conditional on disease status generated from the standard 2-by-2 table

Conditional probabilities	Probability notation	Cell formula
Proportion exposed, given disease	P (E/D)	a/(a + c)
Proportion unexposed, given disease	P (E~/D)	c/(a + c)
Proportion exposed, given nondisease	P (E/D~)	b/(b + d)
Proportion unexposed, given nondisease	P (E~/D~)	d/(b + d)

Quiz 3

Questions 1–12

Researchers gathered data on the relationship between poor reading ability and hypertension. Regarding the 2-by-2 table below, write the answer to each numbered item below.

Table 3-3: Quiz questions on the relationship between reading ability and hypertension

	Hypertension	No hypertension	Total
Poor reading ability	80	20	100
Good reading ability	50	40	90
Total	130	60	190

1. Grand total in the study
2. Number of people who are exposed and diseased
3. Number of people who are unexposed and diseased
4. Number of people who are exposed
5. Number of people who are diseased
6. Proportion (or percentage) exposed and diseased
7. Proportion exposed
8. Proportion nondiseased
9. Proportion diseased, given exposure
10. Proportion nondiseased, given exposure
11. Proportion exposed, given disease
12. Proportion unexposed, given disease

Quiz 3—Answers

1. 190
2. 80
3. 50
4. 100
5. 130
6. 80/190
7. 100/190
8. 60/190
9. 80/100
10. 20/100
11. 80/130
12. 50/130

Lesson 4: The Cross-Sectional Study Design

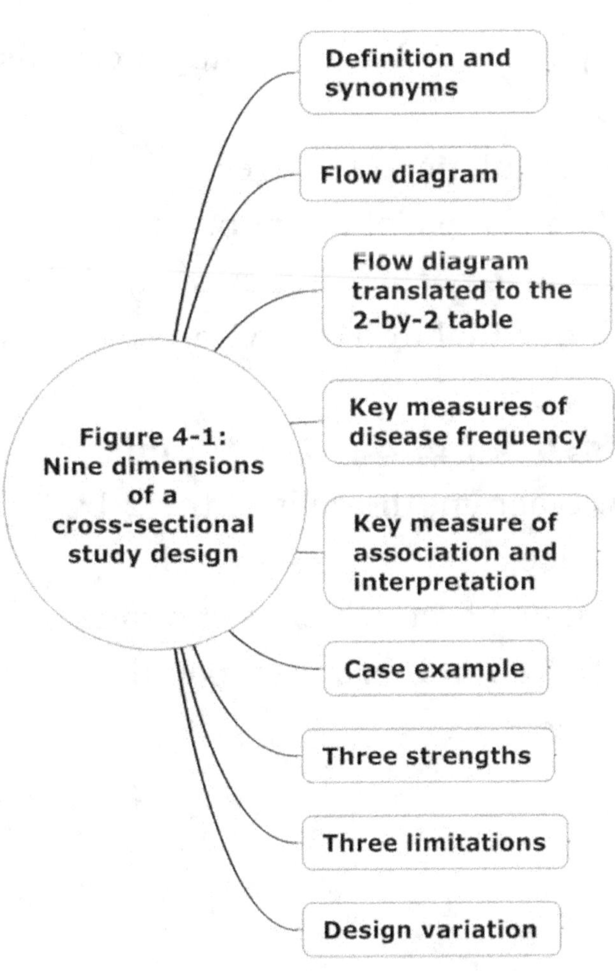

1) Summary

- This lesson covers nine dimensions of the cross-sectional study design (Figure 4-1).

2) Definition and synonyms

I. A **cross-sectional study** is a survey of a population at a *single point in time.*

A. Another name for a cross-sectional study is **prevalence study**.

B. Applications of this study design that you may have heard of include mass screenings, surveys, and opinion polls.

3) Flow diagram

I. There are four steps involved in designing a cross-sectional study (Figure 4-2):

A. Identifying the population of interest

B. Taking a random sample of the population

C. Gathering data on exposure and *existing* disease *simultaneously*

D. Placing each individual into one of four buckets

4) Flow diagram translated to the 2-by-2 table

I. Based on the flow diagram, the cells of the 2-by-2 table are populated in a certain sequence.

A. Cell "n" is populated first, which is the random sample count.

B. Cells "a," "b," "c," and "d" are then populated *simultaneously* (Figure 4-3, Table 3-1).

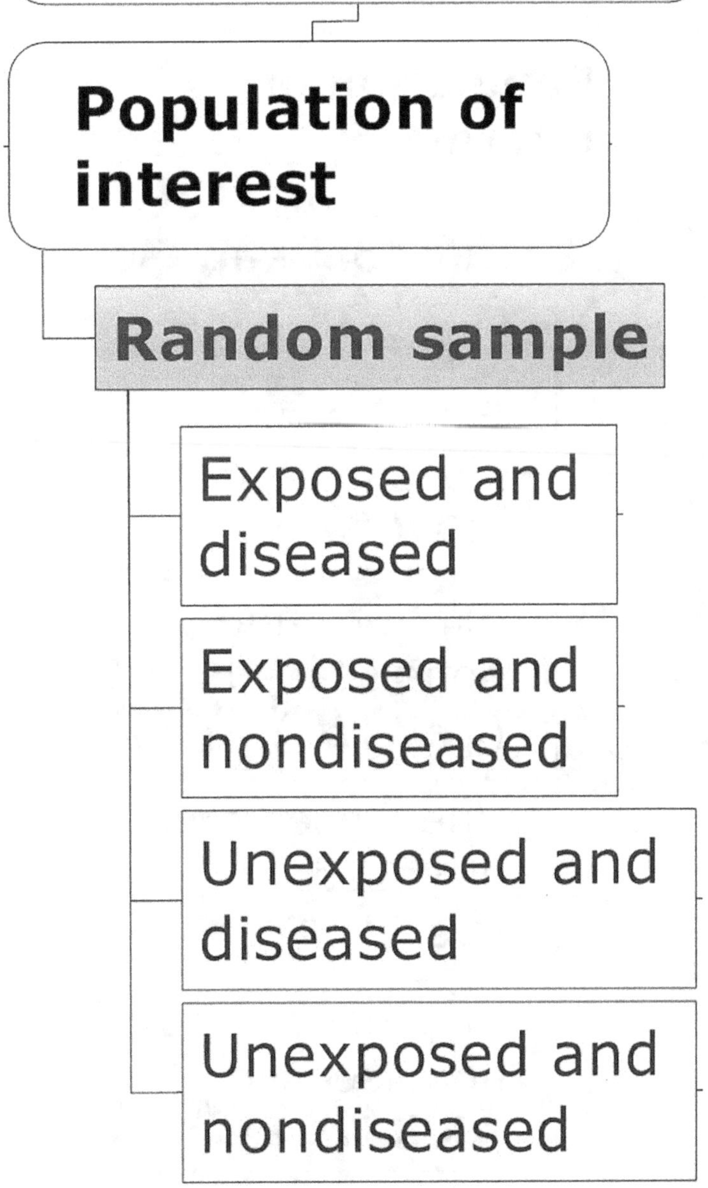

Figure 4-2: Flow diagram of a cross-sectional design

Figure 4-3: Flow diagram of a cross-sectional design, translated to a 2-by-2 table

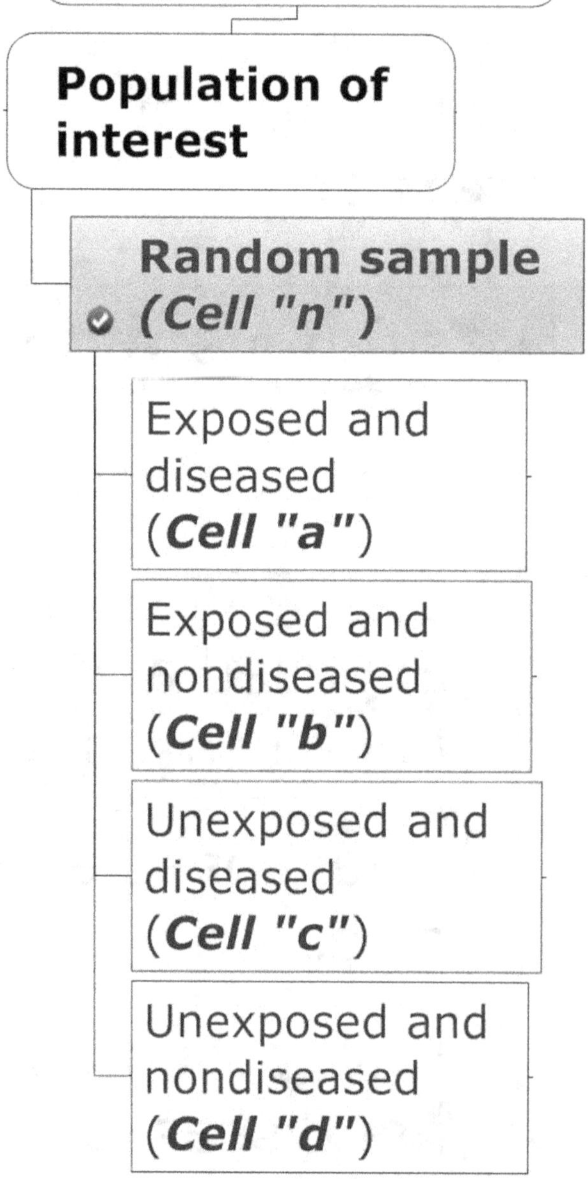

Population of interest

Random sample *(Cell "n")*

Exposed and diseased (***Cell "a"***)

Exposed and nondiseased (***Cell "b"***)

Unexposed and diseased (***Cell "c"***)

Unexposed and nondiseased (***Cell "d"***)

5) Key measures of disease frequency

I. Once study subjects are in their assigned cells, we then calculate the appropriate measures of disease frequency.

A. These measures are based on the **point prevalence**, which is defined as the percentage of the population having the disease or condition of interest at one point in time.

B. There are four key measures of disease frequency (Figure 4-3, Table 3-2B)

1. **Point prevalence of exposure** [(a + b)/n]
2. **Point prevalence of non-exposure** [(c + d)/n]
3. **Point prevalence of disease** [(a + c)/n]
4. **Point prevalence of non-disease** [(b + d)/n]

6) Key measure of association and interpretation

I. Next, we want to calculate the key measure of association, which is the **prevalence ratio** (PR).

A. It is defined as the point prevalence of disease in the exposed group [a/ (a + b)], divided by the point prevalence of disease in the unexposed group [c / (c + d)]. See Table 3-2C.

B. If the PR is greater than 1.0, then the exposed group has a higher point prevalence of disease than the unexposed group. In other words, being in the exposed group is a **risk factor** for disease.

C. If the PR is less than 1.0, then the exposed group has a lower point prevalence of disease than the unexposed group. In other words, being in the exposed group is a **protective factor** against disease.

D. If the PR is equal to 1.0, then the exposed group has a point prevalence of disease equal to that of the unexposed group. In other words, there is no relationship between the exposure and disease.

7) Case example

I. Investigators hypothesized that smoking is positively associated with anxiety. Using a cross-sectional study, 1,000 women were classified according to smoking status and current level of anxiety (Table 4-1).

Table 4-1: Case example of a cross-sectional study

	High anxiety level	Low anxiety level	Totals
Smoker	200	300	500
Nonsmoker	100	400	500
Totals	300	700	1000

A. The point prevalence of smoking is 500/1,000 = 50%.

B. The point prevalence of nonsmoking is 500/1,000 = 50%.

C. The point prevalence of a high anxiety level is 300/1,000 = 30%.

D. The point prevalence of a low anxiety level is 700/1,000 = 70%.

E. The point prevalence of a high anxiety level among smokers is 200/500 = 40%.

F. The point prevalence of a high anxiety level among nonsmokers is 100/500 = 20%.

G. The PR is 40%/20% = 2.

H. The PR is interpreted to mean that smokers are 2 times as likely to have a high anxiety level, compared to nonsmokers. In other words, smoking is a risk factor for a high anxiety level.

I. The hypothesis was supported by the data.

8) Cross-sectional studies have at least three limitations and three strengths

I. Three strengths
  A. First, they provide a "snapshot" of the health experience of a population at a certain point in time.
  B. Second, they can be done quickly and inexpensively because there is no follow-up of study subjects over time.
  C. Third, one can examine relationships among multiple exposures and diseases concurrently.

II. Three limitations
  A. First, there is the **chicken-or-egg dilemma**, also known as **antecedent-consequence uncertainty**.
    1. It is defined as an ambiguous temporal relationship between the exposure and disease. In other words, the fact that the exposure preceded the disease cannot be firmly established because one collected exposure and disease information at the same time.
      a) Referring to the previous case example, we can't be truly certain whether smoking is a risk factor for anxiety or whether anxiety is a risk factor for smoking.
      b) Consider another example of a cross-sectional study exploring the relationship between alcohol use and depression.
        (1) Investigators find that alcohol drinkers are five times as likely to have depression as nondrinkers (PR = 5).
        (2) But, they don't know if alcohol use influences depression or if depression influences alcohol use.
  B. A second disadvantage is that diseases of short duration (quick recovery or quick death) may be under-represented.
    1. That is, one wouldn't get many people in the "D = 1" column of the 2-by-2 table (Table 3-1) because cross-sectional studies provide only a "snapshot" of a population at a certain point in time.

C. A third disadvantage is that it identifies **prevalent** (old and new) cases of disease, not **incident** (new) cases of disease over a follow-up period; and incident cases are required to establish **etiology** (formally linking a factor to the *initiation* of disease).

9) Design Variation

- There are no design variations.

Quiz 4

Procedural knowledge

Questions 1–9
The Faulkner Foundation has asked communities to submit proposals that request funds for programs to reduce race gaps in physical assault. To be considered for funding, however, a community must first present data in its proposal that show that a racial disparity exists in that community. Seminole County, Florida, decides to apply for funding. They identify data from a cross-sectional study conducted in their county. The 2-by-2 table is set up like this:

E is "African-American (AA) women"
E~ is "white (W) women"
D is "physical assault"
D~ is "no physical assault"
Cell a = 200
Cell b = 800
Cell c = 100
Cell d = 900

1. What is the overall point prevalence of physical assault among these women?

   A. 200/1,000
   B. 100/1,000
   C. 300/2,000
   D. 300/1,700

2. What is the overall point prevalence of no physical assault among these women?

   A. 1,700/2,000
   B. 1,000/2,000
   C. 300/2,000
   D. 300/1,700

3. What is the point prevalence of exposure (being African-American)?

   A. 1,700/2,000
   B. 1,000/2,000
   C. 300/2,000
   D. 300/1,700

4. What is the point prevalence of nonexposure (being white)?

   A. 1,700/2,000
   B. 1,000/2,000
   C. 300/2,000
   D. 300/1,700

5. What is the point prevalence of physical assault among AA women?

   A. 200/1,000
   B. 200/800
   C. 200/300
   D. 200/100

6. What is the point prevalence of physical assault among W women?

   A. 100/1,000
   B. 100/900
   C. 100/300
   D. 100/200

7. What is the prevalence ratio (PR) of physical assault for AA women compared to W women?

   A. 0.5
   B. 0.4
   C. 2.0
   D. 2.3

8. Is Seminole County eligible for funding consideration? That is, in Seminole County, are AA women more likely to suffer from physical assaults than W women?

   A. Yes
   B. No
   C. That cannot be determined from these data.

9. If the PR above were 3.0, how would it be interpreted?

   A. The prevalence of physical assault among white women is 3 times the prevalence of physical assault among African-American women.
   B. The prevalence of physical assault among African-American women is 3 times the prevalence of physical assault among white women.
   C. White race is a risk factor for physical assault.
   D. African-American race is a risk factor for physical assault.
   E. A and C
   F. B and D

Declarative knowledge

10. Antecedent-consequence uncertainty is defined as:

   A. A form of bias occurring when the level of uncertainty associated with the measurement of the outcome (consequence) differs for cases and controls.
   B. A form of bias resulting from a statistically insignificant increase in the occurrence of the outcome (consequence) as a result of exposure (antecedent).
   C. A form of bias resulting from confusion as to whether the exposure precedes or follows an outcome.
   D. A form of bias in which the antecedent is more likely to precede the consequence in cases than in controls.

11. In a large cross-sectional study, 10 of every 100,000 African-American men are found to have prostate cancer compared to 20 out of every 100,000 white men. The epidemiologist conducting the study concludes that white men have a higher likelihood of developing prostate cancer. This conclusion is:

    A. Correct for this study population.
    B. Incorrect because of failure to distinguish between prevalent cases and incident cases.
    C. Incorrect because only men were studied, therefore the study lacks an appropriate control group.
    D. Incorrect if there are more white men than African-American men in the study population.

Quiz 4: Answers

1. C
2. A
3. B
4. B
5. A
6. A
7. C; answer #5 above divided by answer #6 above = 2.0
8. A
9. F
10. C
11. B; the conclusion should be that white men have a higher likelihood of *having* prostate cancer; "having" indicates prevalent cases, while "developing" indicates incident cases.

Lesson 5: The Population-Based Prospective Cohort Study Design

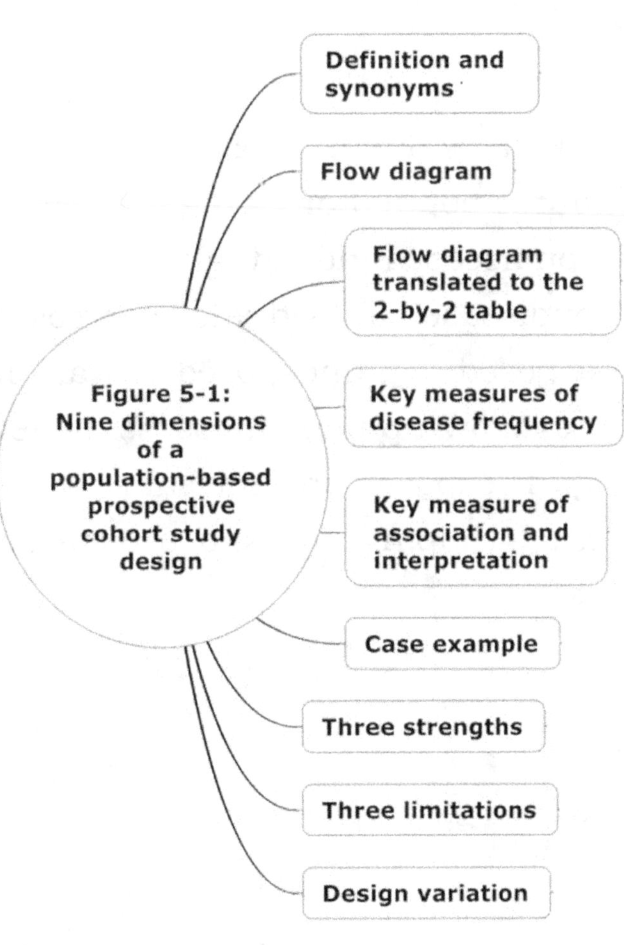

1) Summary

- This lesson describes the population-based prospective cohort study design, with respect to the nine dimensions (Figure 5-1).

2) Definition and synonyms

I. In **prospective cohort studies**, subjects are characterized by exposure level in the present and are then followed forward in time to assess the development of a condition.

A. Other names for this study design include **follow-up study**, **incidence study**, and **longitudinal study**.

II. In a ***population-based*** prospective cohort study, all of the study subjects come from the same geographically defined **source population** (such as Framingham, Massachusetts).

3) Flow diagram

I. There are five design steps (Figure 5-2):

A. Selecting the source population

B. Screening for nondiseased individuals

C. Labeling the nondiseased individuals as exposed or unexposed

D. Following the exposed and unexposed forward in time

E. At the end of the follow-up period, assessing new disease status (yes, no) among the exposed and the same among the unexposed

II. In summary, we are "grouping" by exposure status and then "assessing" disease status.

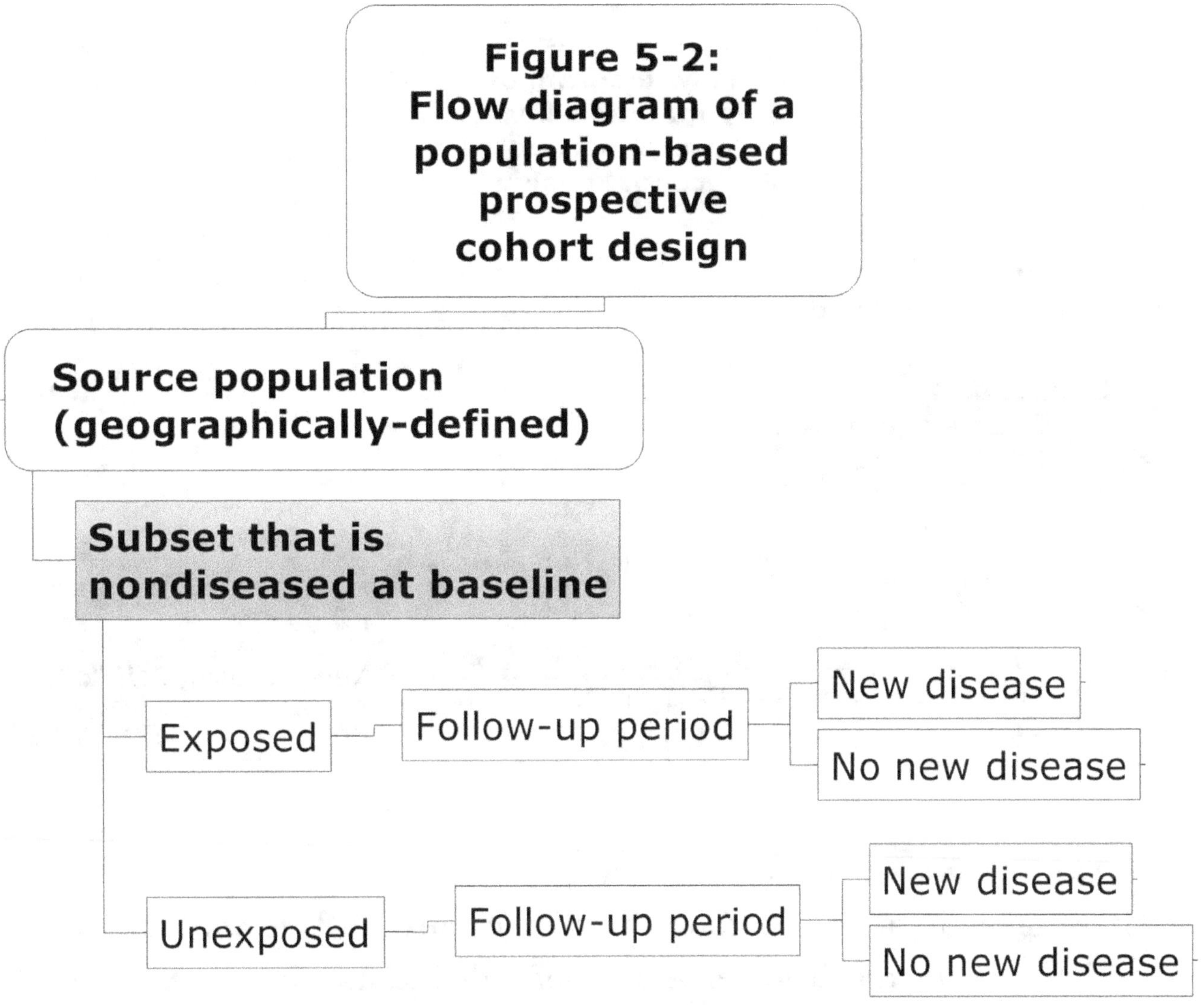

4) Flow diagram translated to the 2-by-2 table

I. Based on the flow diagram, the cells of the 2-by-2 table are populated in a certain sequence.

II. Cell "n" is populated first.

III. Next, cells "a + b" and "c + d," the row marginal totals (Lesson 3), are populated.

IV. Finally, after the follow-up period, the values of cells "a," "b," "c," and "d" become known (Figure 5-3, Table 3-1).

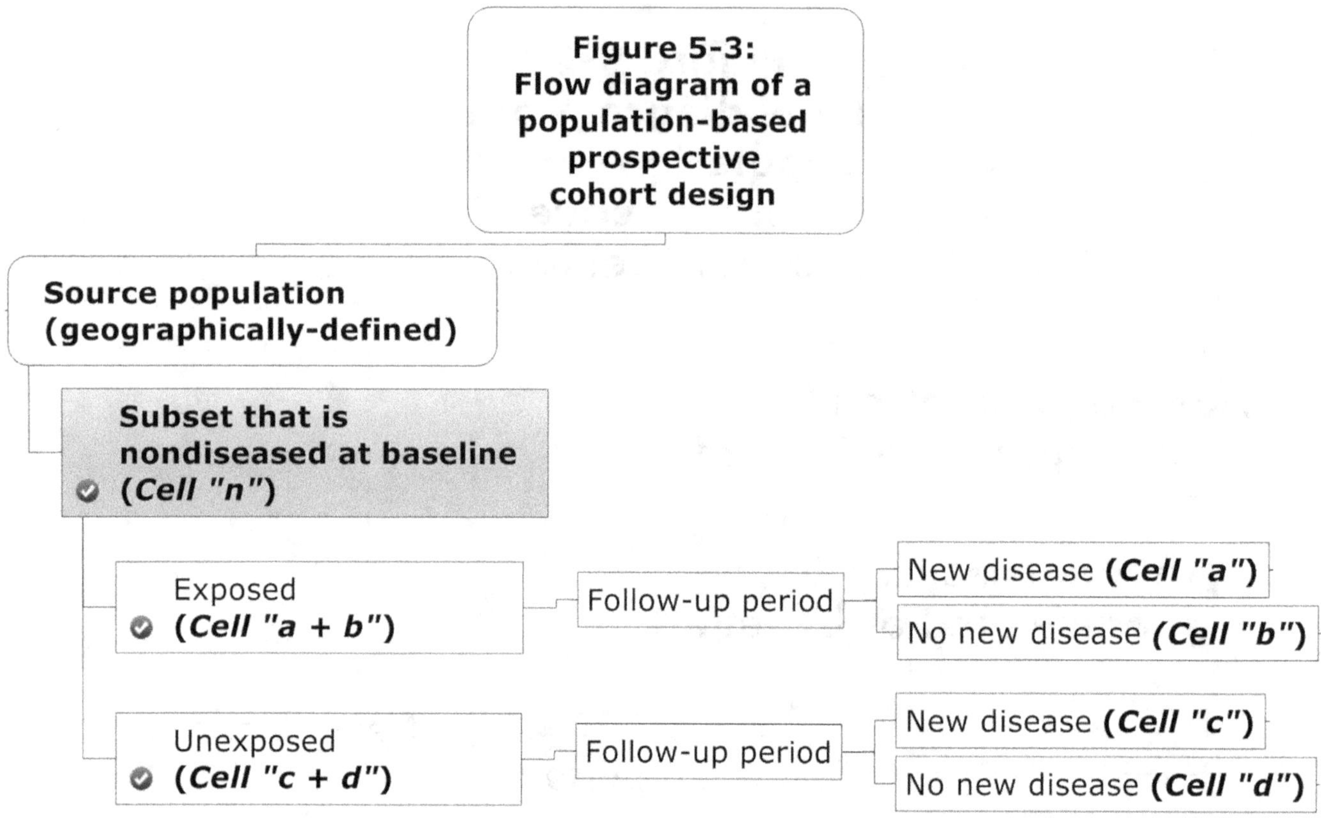

5) Key measures of disease frequency

I. These measures are based on the **risk** (or **cumulative incidence**), which is defined as the percentage of individuals who *develop* the event during a period of time.

A. There are two key measures of disease frequency (Figure 5-3, Table 3-2C)

1. **Risk of disease in the exposed** [a/ (a + b)]
2. **Risk of disease in the unexposed** [c/ (c + d)]

6) Key measure of association and interpretation

I. The key measure of association is the **risk ratio** (RR).

   A. It is defined as the risk of disease in the exposed group [a/ (a + b)] divided by the risk of disease in the unexposed group [c/ (c + d)]. (Please see Figure 5-3 and Table 3-2C.)

   B. Notice that the letter-formula for the RR is the same as the letter-formula for the PR (Lesson 4); however, the RR refers to *new* cases of disease, while the PR refers to *existing* cases of disease.

II. If the RR is greater than 1.0, then the exposed group has a higher risk of disease than the unexposed group. In other words, being in the exposed group is a risk factor for disease.

III. If the RR is less than 1.0, then the exposed group has a lower risk of disease than the unexposed group. In other words, being in the exposed group is a protective factor against disease.

IV. If the RR is equal to 1.0, then the exposed group has a risk equal to that of the unexposed group. In other words, there is no relationship between the exposure and disease.

7) Case example

I. A cohort study is conducted, hypothesizing the positive association between dietary fat intake and the development of prostate cancer (CA) in men. In the study, 100 men with a high-fat diet are compared with 100 men who are on a low-fat diet. Both groups start at age 65 and are followed for 10 years. During the follow-up period, 10 men in the high-fat intake group are diagnosed with prostate cancer and 5 men in the low-fat intake group develop prostate cancer (Table 5-1).

Table 5-1: Case example of a population-based prospective cohort study

	Cancer	No cancer	Total
High-fat diet	10	90	100
Low-fat diet	5	95	100
Total	15	185	200

A. The risk of developing prostate CA in the high-fat group is 10/100 = 10% over 10 years.

B. The risk of developing prostate CA in the low-fat group is 5/100 = 5% over 10 years.

C. The risk ratio is 10%/ 5% = 2.

D. Those with a high-fat diet are 2 times as likely to develop prostate cancer as those on a low-fat diet. In other words, a high-fat diet is a risk factor for prostate cancer in men.

E. The hypothesis was supported by the data.

8) Three strengths and three limitations

I. Strengths

A. First, unlike a cross-sectional design (Lesson 4), the population-based prospective cohort design identifies incident (new) cases of disease over a follow-up period. (Recall that incident cases are required for formal establishment of etiology.)

B. Second, unlike with a cross-sectional design, there is no antecedent-consequence bias. That is, we know that the exposure preceded disease because of the flow diagram (Figure 5-2).

C. Third, the investigator is able to take time to measure the exposure variable (for example, dietary habits) accurately and completely. He or she is also able to control and standardize data collection as the study progresses.

II. Limitations

A. First, one needs a large number of subjects with the potential to develop the disease of interest over a period of time; therefore, it is expensive.

B. Second, follow-up periods can be lengthy and time-consuming.

C. Third, there could be **losses to follow-up**.

1. More specifically, there may be attrition of the cohort during the follow-up period because of migration, lack of participation, or death from diseases other than the disease of interest.
2. The significance is that you don't know whether lost individuals would have developed the disease of interest or not.

9) Design variation

I. In a prospective cohort design, nondiseased individuals are grouped by exposure status at **baseline** (*the present*) and then followed into the future for the occurrence of new disease.

A. Depending on the size of the cohort and the prevalence of disease in the population, several years could pass before meaningful analyses are feasible.

II. An alternative is the **retrospective cohort study design**.

A. The retrospective cohort study makes use of historical data to determine exposure level at some baseline in the *past*.

B. Follow-up for disease occurrence takes place between baseline and the present (Figure 5-4).

C. This study design is also referred to as an **historical cohort design** or a **nonconcurrent cohort design**.

D. The key measures of disease frequency and key measure of association for the retrospective cohort design are the same as those of the prospective cohort design.

   1. As an example, consider that in 2001 investigators initiated a study to examine the relationship between neonatal asphyxia and intellectual functioning.

      a) Exposure status was determined by medical record reviews of infants born in a certain hospital in 1989.

      b) Disease status was determined by a review of school achievement records from 1999–2000.

E. Compared to prospective cohort designs, retrospective designs have at least two strengths.

   1. They take less time and money because all relevant exposure and disease events have already occurred at the start of the study.

   2. Therefore, they are particularly efficient for diseases with long **latency periods** (the period between the onset of a cause and disease appearance or detection).

F. On the other hand, compared to prospective cohort designs, retrospective designs have at least two limitations.

   1. First, investigators depend on pre-existing records for exposure and disease information.

      a) These records were not likely designed for research purposes.

      b) Therefore, they may be incomplete and noncomparable across all study subjects.

2. Second, pre-existing records tend not to have information on **confounding variables** (variables other than the exposure and disease variables that may influence the results).

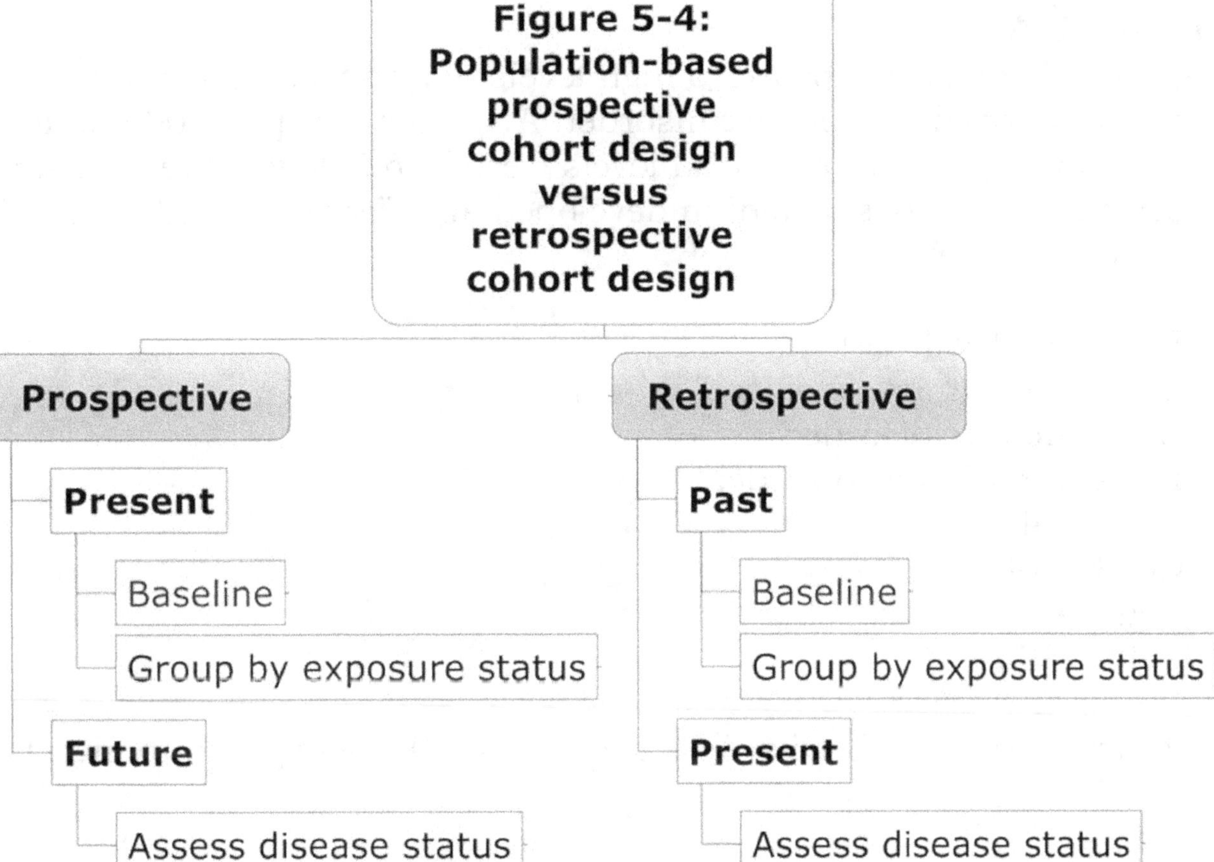

Quiz 5

Procedural knowledge

Questions 1–4

One hundred children exposed to high levels of lead were followed for 15 years; 40 developed an affective disorder. A similar group of 100 children who were not exposed to high lead levels were also followed over the same time period. Five of these children developed an affective disorder. The data are summarized below.

E is "high levels of lead"
E~ is "no high levels of lead"
D is "affective disorder"
D~ is "no affective disorder"
Cell a = 40
Cell b = 60
Cell c = 5
Cell d = 95

1. What is the risk of affective disorders among those exposed to high levels of lead?

   A. 0.20
   B. 0.05
   C. 0.40
   D. 0.225

2. What is the risk of affective disorders among those not exposed to high levels of lead?

   A. 0.20
   B. 0.05
   C. 0.40
   D. 0.225

3. What is the relative risk (RR) of developing an affective disorder for those exposed to high levels of lead compared to those with no such exposure?

    A. 12.67
    B. 8.0
    C. 0.23
    D. 0.40

4. What overall conclusion can we draw from the RR?

    A. High lead exposure is a risk factor for affective disorders
    B. High lead exposure is a protective factor against affective disorders
    C. There is no relationship between high lead exposure and affective disorders
    D. We can't draw a conclusion because the RR can't be calculated

Declarative knowledge

5. A prospective cohort study employs:

    A. Subjects known at the start to have the disease of interest
    B. Subjects known at the start to be disease-free
    C. Subjects whose exposure to a suspected risk factor is comparable to that of the control group at the start of the study
    D. Comparison groups of equal size

6. With cohort studies, you're "grouping" people based on whether they are _____; and then you're "assessing" people based on whether they are _____.

    A. Exposed or not; diseased or not
    B. Diseased or not; exposed or not

7. Some advantages of cohort studies are that:

   A. They are relatively inexpensive and logistically simple to conduct
   B. They are well-suited for study of rare diseases
   C. Losses to follow-up will not affect study results
   D. Incidence of disease can be measured directly
   E. All of the above
   F. A, B, and C
   G. A and C
   H. B and D

Questions 8–14
Instructions: For each numbered study characteristic below, choose the most appropriate lettered answer. A given letter may be used once, more than once, or not at all.

Lettered response options:

A. Both prospective and retrospective cohort studies
B. Neither prospective nor retrospective cohort study
C. Prospective cohort study
D. Retrospective cohort study

8. Less expensive

9. Quicker

10. More accurate exposure information

11. Better for studying the effects of discontinued exposures

12. Appropriate for studying rare diseases

13. Problems with loss to follow-up

14. Better for diseases with long latency periods

Quiz 5–Answers

1. C; 40/ (40 + 60) = 40/100 = 0.40
2. B; 5/(5 + 95) = 5/100 = 0.05
3. B; answer #1 above divided by answer #2 above = 8.0
4. A
5. B
6. A
7. D
8. D; a comparison between the retrospective and prospective designs is implied by the word, "less"
9. D; a comparison between the retrospective and prospective designs is implied by the word, "quicker"
10. C; a comparison between the retrospective and prospective designs is implied by the word, "more"
11. D; a comparison between the retrospective and prospective designs is implied by the word, "better"
12. B
13. A
14. D; a comparison between the retrospective and prospective designs is implied by the word, "better"

Lesson 6: The Population-Based Case-Control Study Design

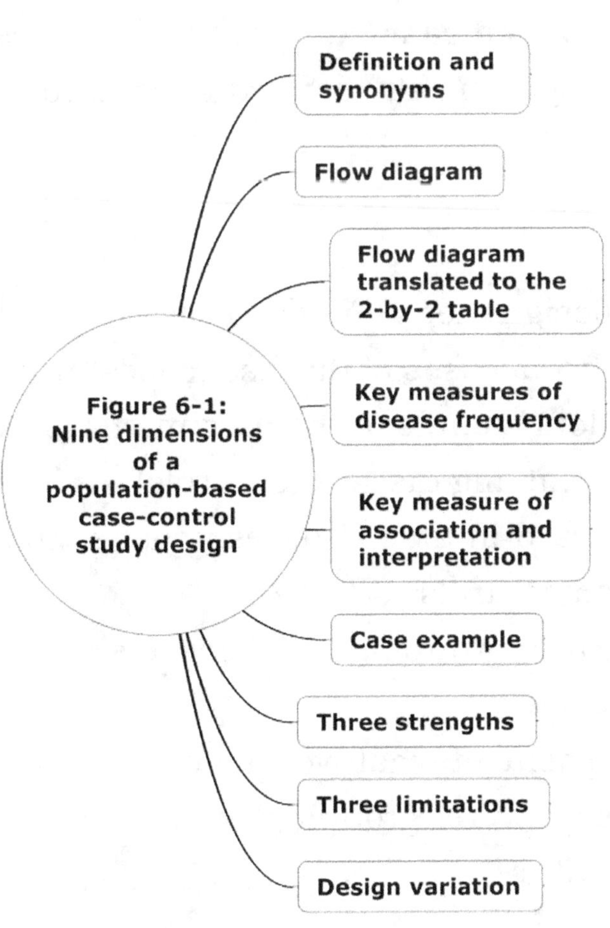

1) Summary

- This lesson describes the population-based case-control study design from the perspective of nine dimensions (Figure 6-1).

2) Definition and synonyms

I. In a **case-control study**, the investigator identifies one group with the disease (**cases**) and another without it (**controls**) and then looks *backward* to find differences in suspected exposures that may explain why the cases got the disease and the controls did not.

   A. The case-control design is considered "**retrospective**" because, conceptually, it goes from disease onset backward to the suspected exposures.

   B. A synonym for a case-control study is "**case-referent study.**"

II. In a ***population-based*** **case-control study**, cases and controls come from the same geographically defined source population, known as the **catchment area**.

3) Flow diagram

I. There are three design steps (Figure 6-2):

   A. Identifying *all new* cases of disease (cases) from a catchment area

   B. Taking a random sample of the catchment area and identifying those with no existing disease (controls)

   C. Looking backward in time to assess past exposure status among both cases and controls

II. In summary, we are "grouping by" disease status and then "assessing" exposure status.

   A. This is the opposite of what we saw with the prospective cohort design, where we were "grouping" by exposure status then "assessing" disease status.

III. Why do we want to identify *new* cases of disease?
   A. Incident (new) cases are preferable to prevalent (old and new) cases.
      1. One reason is that disease diagnostic methods change over time, so recent diagnoses are more likely to be homogeneous.
      2. Secondly, individuals with new disease will remember their past exposure history better than individuals with prevalent disease.
      3. Thirdly, there is a reduced likelihood that the exposure has changed as a *consequence* of the disease.
      4. Finally, incident cases are required for establishing etiology.

IV. Why do we want to identify *all* new cases of disease?
   A. If we have only *some* of the new cases in our study, we wonder whether our cases are adequately representative of all those with incident disease.

V. Why are we interested in *past* (versus current) exposure status?
   A. If we study past exposure history and incident disease, then we are more confident that the exposure preceded the disease. In other words, we are minimizing antecedent-consequence bias.

VI. *Where* can we find all new cases of disease?
   A. One ideal source is the **population-based disease registry**, which provides a listing of all new cases of a disease or health-related condition in a geographic area.
      1. For example, registries exist for new cases of birth defects, AIDS, and sudden infant death.
      2. The **Surveillance Epidemiology and End Results (SEER)** program is a coalition of population-based cancer registries.

VII. How do we find appropriate controls?
   A. If cases come from a population-based disease registry, then a representative sample of the population living in the area (catchment area) covered by the registry would be the control group (Figure 6-2).

B. Area tax lists, voting lists, and telephone directories may be useful rosters from which samples can be drawn, provided that their coverage of the population is complete or nearly complete.

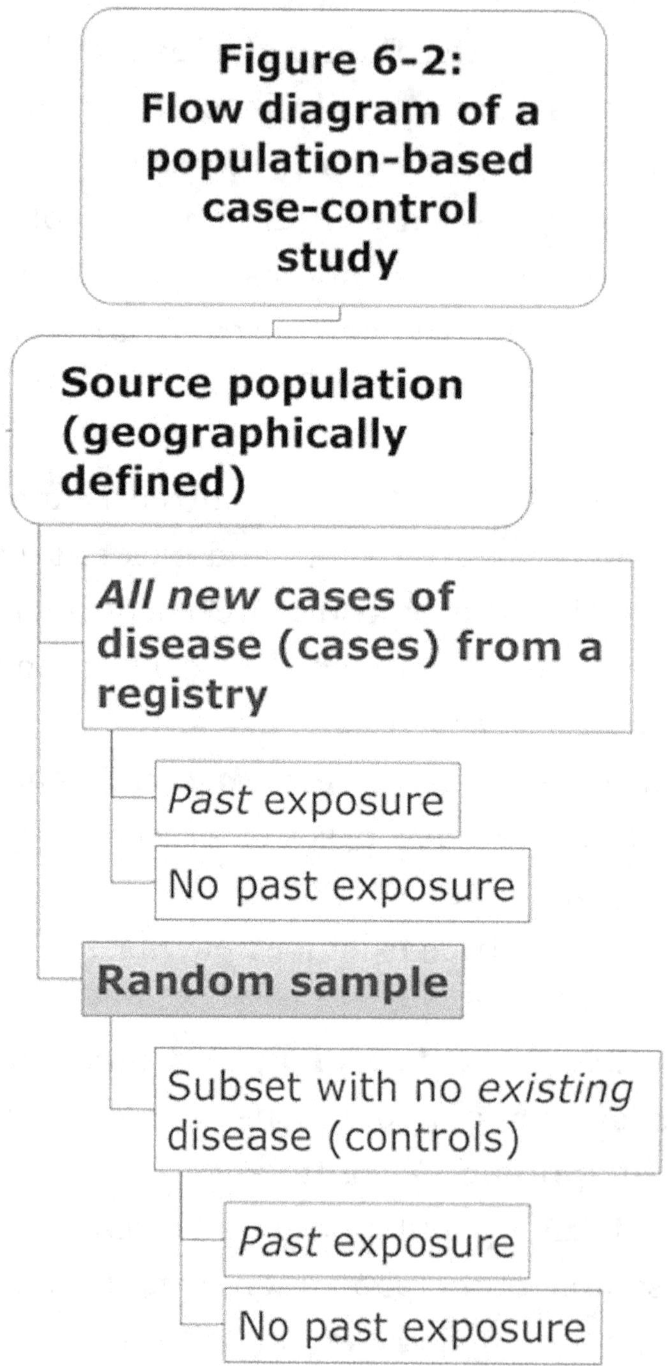

4) *Flow diagram translated to the 2-by-2 table*

I. Based on the flow diagram, the cells of the 2-by-2 table are populated in a certain sequence.
   A. Cells "a + c" and "b + d," the column marginal totals (Lesson 3), are populated first.
   B. Then cells "a," "b," "c," and "d" are populated (Figure 6-3, Table 3-1).

5) *Key measures of disease frequency*

I. There are two key measures of disease frequency: the **odds of exposure among cases** and the **odds of exposure among controls**.
   A. The **odds** are the percentage experiencing an event divided by the percentage not experiencing the event.
   B. Since we are grouping by disease status and *assessing* exposure status, the "event" here is exposure (E = 1). See Table 3-1.
   C. Thus, among cases the odds of exposure = [a/ (a + c)] divided by [c/ (a + c)]. This expression simplifies to a/c. See Table 3-2D.
   D. Among controls the odds of exposure = [b/ (b + d)] divided by [d/ (b +d)]. This expression simplifies to b/d. See Table 3-2D.

6) *Key measure of association and interpretation*

I. The key measure of association is the **exposure odds ratio** (EOR).
   A. It is defined as the odds of exposure in the cases (a/c) divided by the odds of exposure in the controls (b/d).
   B. If the EOR is greater than 1.0, then cases have a higher odds of exposure than controls. In other words, exposure is a risk factor for disease.
   C. If the EOR is less than 1.0, then cases have a lower odds of exposure than controls. In other words, exposure is a protective factor against disease.
   D. If the EOR is equal to 1.0, then cases have an odds of exposure equal to that of controls. In other words, there is no relationship between the exposure and disease.

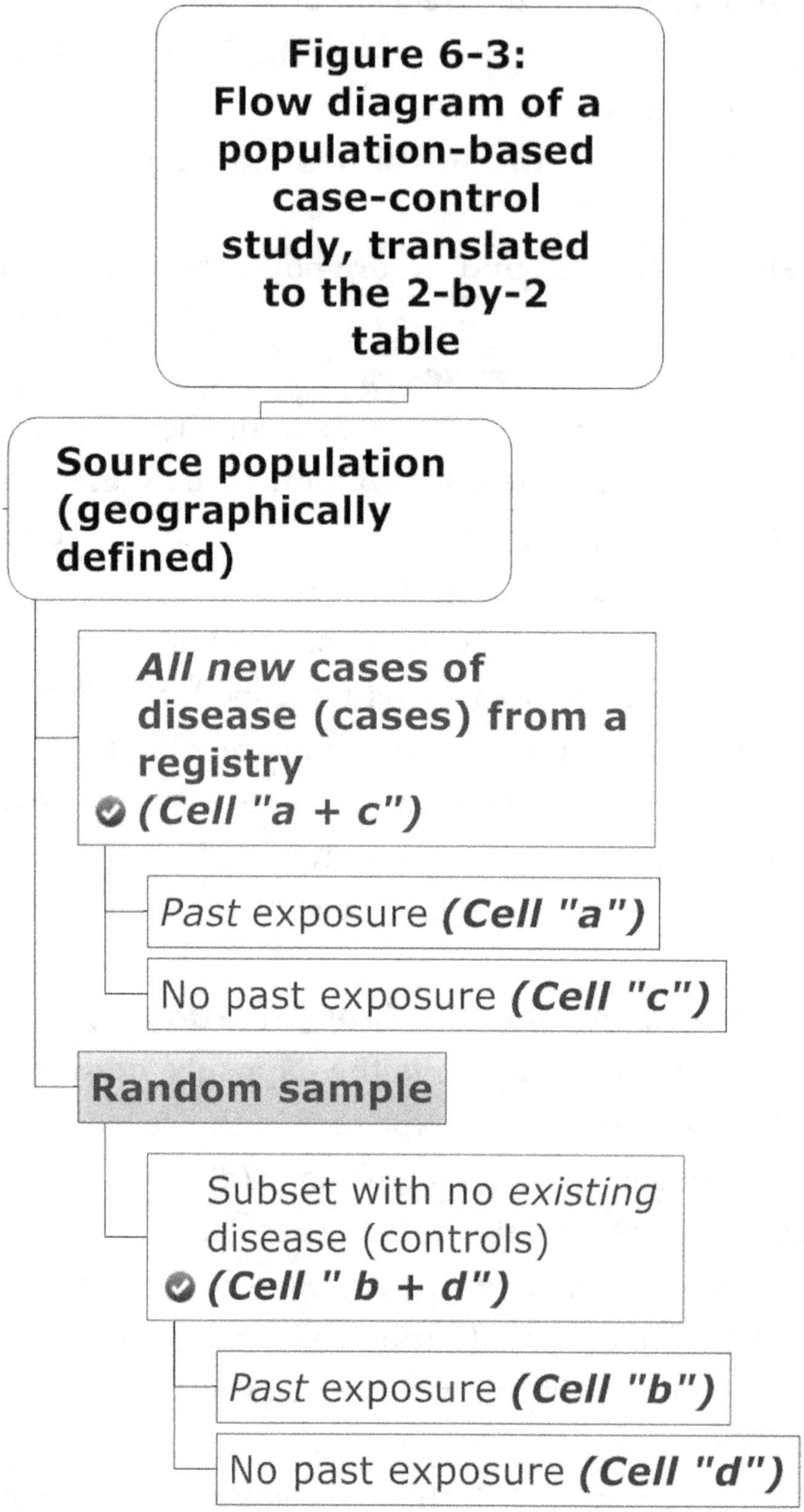

Figure 6-3: Flow diagram of a population-based case-control study, translated to the 2-by-2 table

Source population (geographically defined)

- ***All new*** **cases of disease (cases) from a registry** ***(Cell "a + c")***
  - *Past* exposure ***(Cell "a")***
  - No past exposure ***(Cell "c")***
- **Random sample**
  - Subset with no *existing* disease (controls) ***(Cell " b + d")***
    - *Past* exposure ***(Cell "b")***
    - No past exposure ***(Cell "d")***

7) Case example

I. In Mexico City, a population-based case-control study was conducted hypothesizing the positive association between chili pepper consumption and gastric cancer. Subjects consisted of 213 incident cases and 697 controls that were randomly selected from the general population. Interviews produced information regarding chili pepper consumption (Table 6-1).

Table 6-1: Case example of a population-based case-control study

	Cancer	No Cancer	Total
Chili peppers	204	552	756
No chili peppers	9	145	154
Total	213	697	910

A. The odds of chili pepper consumption among cases = 204/9 = 22.67.

B. The odds of chili pepper consumption among controls = 552/145 = 3.81.

C. The exposure odds ratio (EOR) = 22.67/3.81 = 5.95.

D. Thus, gastric cancer cases have 5.95 times the odds of chili pepper consumption compared to controls. In other words, chili pepper consumption is a risk factor for gastric cancer.

E. The hypothesis was supported by the data.

8) Three strengths and three limitations

I. There are at least three advantages of this study design.

A. First, it is quicker and less expensive than prospective cohort studies because there is no follow-up period.

B. Second, it is efficient for investigation of diseases with long latency periods (long intervals between disease initiation and clinical emergence), in which instance a prospective cohort study would involve many years of follow-up before the outcome became evident. Cancers, for instance, tend to have long latency periods.

C. Third, it can evaluate multiple exposures in relation to the same disease, so it is good for diseases about which little is known.

II. There are at least three disadvantages.

A. First, unlike with a prospective cohort study, we cannot *directly* estimate the risk ratio (RR) from the 2-by-2 table. (The RR can be calculated *indirectly* via a series of equations using information external to the study, but these computations are outside the scope of this book.)

1. This is because in a 2-by-2 table of a case-control study, the column totals of diseased and nondiseased individuals are prefixed by the investigator prior to the start of the study.
2. Therefore, measures of disease frequency based upon the probability (%) of disease (Table 3-2C) cannot be estimated with this study design. (RR = % diseased in the exposed group/ % diseased in the unexposed group.)

B. Second, because of the retrospective nature of the design, antecedent-consequence uncertainty may occur.

C. Third, there is a possibility of **recall bias**.

1. Recall bias is systematic error due to differences in accuracy or completeness of recall of past events or experiences.

a) For example, say that we conducted a study on the association between over-the-counter (OTC) medication use and birth defects.

(1) Cases are defined as mothers of infants born with birth defects.

(2) Controls are defined as mothers of normal infants.

(3) Both groups are asked about their past OTC medication use during pregnancy.

(4) Cases will be more likely to overestimate their past OTC medication use than controls. This is because they are ruminating, trying to find an explanation for their infants' birth defects.

(5) In the end, cell "a" of the 2-by-2 table will be larger than it should be, and the EOR will be exaggerated as well.

9) Design variation

I. A **hospital-based case-control design** is one variation of the population-based case-control design. In the hospital-based variation, the cases and controls come from the same hospital or hospital network.

A. In a typical design flow, given a hospital admissions database, the investigator:

1. Identifies all persons admitted to a hospital with the recently diagnosed condition of interest (cases)
2. Selects all persons admitted to the same hospital with another recently diagnosed condition but with no evidence of the condition of interest (controls)
3. Obtains information about past exposure from cases and controls, often by interviewing them in the hospital

B. For example, investigators conducted a hospital-based case-control study on risks for spontaneous abortion.
   1. Women who experienced a pregnancy loss (cases) were identified each weekday from hospital admissions records, and they were interviewed about their prior exposures before hospital discharge.
   2. Women who delivered live-born infants at the same hospital comprised the control group; they were also interviewed about their prior exposures before hospital discharge.

C. The key measures of disease frequency and the key measure of association for the hospital-based design are the same as those of their population-based counterpart.

D. There are at least two advantages of the hospital-based design compared to the population-based design.
   1. First, subjects tend to be more cooperative because they are ill and may want to advance medical knowledge.
   2. Second, it is easier to collect exposure information (e.g., from medical records, biological specimens, or interviews) in a hospital environment.

E. On the other hand, there are at least two disadvantages of the hospital-based design compared to its population-based counterpart.
   1. First, cases and controls may not come from the same, single, well-defined source population.
      a) This could happen when the hospital sees patients from multiple geographic areas, and the areas vary by disease diagnosis.
      b) Different source populations are problematic because differences in unmeasured factors interfere with validly computing the EORs.

2. Second, hospital controls do have a condition, and the exposure of interest may be a risk factor for the control-condition (condition "Y"), as well as the case-condition (condition "X").
   a) For example, early case-control studies of smoking and lung cancer selected controls from patients with diseases other than lung cancer.
      (1) It was not recognized that smoking is a risk factor for a wide range of disease conditions that result in hospitalization.
      (2) As a result, the deleterious (or harmful) effect of smoking on lung cancer was diluted or underestimated.
      (3) Under some circumstances, the exposure of interest may be a *protective factor* for condition "Y" and condition "X." Here, the protective effect is diluted.

Quiz 6

Procedural knowledge

Questions 1–5

In a case-control study examining the relationship between developmental disorders and prenatal exposure to cocaine, the hospital records of 1,000 infants diagnosed with a developmental disorder and 1,000 control infants were inspected for proven maternal cocaine abuse.

E is "prenatal cocaine use"
E~ is "no prenatal cocaine use"
D is "developmental disorder"
D~ is "no developmental disorder"
Cell a = 800
Cell b = 300
Cell c = 200
Cell d = 700

1. What are the exposure odds for cases?

A. (800/1,000) / (200/1,000) = 800/200
B. 800/1,000
C. (300/1,000) / (700/1,000) = 300/700
D. 300/1000
E. Cannot be computed from the data

2. What are the exposure odds for controls?

A. (800/1,000) / (200/1,000) = 800/200
B. 800/1,000
C. (300/1,000) / (700/1,000) = 300/700
D. 300/1,000
E. Cannot be computed from the data

3. What is the value of the exposure odds ratio (EOR)?

   A. 9.33
   B. 3.27
   C. 0.73
   D. 0.80

4. What general conclusion can we draw?

   A. Developmental disorders are a risk factor for prenatal cocaine use.
   B. Developmental disorders are a protective factor against prenatal cocaine use.
   C. Prenatal cocaine use is a risk factor for developmental disorders.
   D. Prenatal cocaine use is a protective factor against developmental disorders.
   E. There is no statistical relationship between prenatal cocaine use and developmental disorders.

5. If the value of the odds ratio were 5.0, how would it be literally interpreted?

   A. The odds of having a developmental disorder are 5 times higher among those with prenatal cocaine exposure than those without prenatal cocaine exposure.
   B. The odds of prenatal cocaine exposure are 5 times higher among those with developmental disorders than those without developmental disorders.
   C. Those with prenatal cocaine exposure are 5 times more likely to have developmental disorders than those without prenatal cocaine exposure.
   D. Those with developmental disorders are 5 times more likely to have had prenatal cocaine exposure than those without developmental disorders.

Declarative knowledge

6. In a case-control study that is being planned to study possible causes of myocardial infarction (heart disease), patients with myocardial infarction serve as the cases. Which of the following would be a poor choice to serve as the controls?

   A. Subjects who have no history of myocardial infarction
   B. Subjects who were admitted to the hospital for noncardiac diseases
   C. Subjects whose age distribution is similar to that of cases
   D. Subjects whose cardiac risk factors are similar to those of cases
   E. Subjects whose socio-demographic characteristics are similar to those of the cases

7. With case-control studies, you are "grouped" based on whether you are____ and "assessed" based on whether you are _____.

   A. Exposed or not; diseased or not
   B. Diseased or not; exposed or not

8. Given a case-control study on the relationship between environmental tobacco smoke (ETS) exposure and asthma, we'd be *assessing* _____ETS exposure not ____ ETS exposure.

   A. Current; past
   B. Past; current

9. A case-control study is characterized by all of the following *except*:

   A. It is relatively inexpensive compared with most other epidemiologic study designs.
   B. Persons with the disease (cases) are compared to persons without the disease (controls).
   C. Incidence measures may be computed directly.
   D. Assessment of past exposure may be biased.
   E. Definition of cases may be difficult.

10. In a case-control study, which of the following is true?

    A. To some extent, the proportion of cases with the exposure is compared with the proportion of controls with the exposure.
    B. Disease percentages are compared for people with the exposure of interest and for people without the exposure of interest.
    C. Recall bias is a potential problem.
    D. A and C

Quiz 6–Answers

1. A
2. C
3. A; answer #1 above divided by answer #2 above = 9.33
4. C
5. B
6. D
7. B
8. B
9. C
10. D

Lesson 7: Book Summary Materials

1) Summary

- Please study Figure 7-1 and Worksheet 7-1 (both located at the end of this chapter).
- Then, take the comprehensive exam below.
- The answer key follows the exam.

2) Comprehensive Exam

Questions 1–10

For each numbered item, choose the most appropriate lettered, study design name. A given letter may be used once, more than once, or not at all.

Lettered response options (Questions 1-10, next page):

A. Cross-sectional study
B. Prospective cohort study
C. Retrospective cohort study
D. Case-control study

1. Case-referent study

2. Mass screenings

3. Opinion polls

4. Prevalence ratio

5. Surveys

6. Prevalence study

7. Point prevalence of exposure

8. Nonconcurrent cohort design

9. Historical cohort design

10. Exposure odds ratio

Lettered response options (Questions 1-10):
A. Cross-sectional study
B. Prospective cohort study
C. Retrospective cohort study
D. Case-control study

Questions 11–15

For each numbered study characteristic below, choose the most appropriate lettered answer. A given letter may be used once, more than once, or not at all.

Lettered response options: (Questions 11-15):
A. Prospective cohort study
B. Retrospective cohort study
C. Case-control study
D. Cross-sectional study

11. Best for identifying *causes* of a *rare disease*

12. Best for identifying the *long-term* health effects of a *rare exposure*

13. Best for identifying the *causes* of a *new disease* about which little is known

14. Best for identifying the *short-term* health effects of a *new exposure* about which little is known

15. Best for identifying the *causes* of a disease with a *long latency period*

16. A conceptual hypothesis states that the dependent variable decreases as the independent variable decreases. This hypothesis is indicating a/an:

    A. Positive association
    B. Negative (or inverse) association
    C. Null association

17. If a categorical variable's response options cover the entire realm of possible answers ("no gaps"), then the response options are ______

    A. Mutually exclusive
    B. Exhaustive

18. If a categorical variable's response options do not overlap each other ("no overlaps"), then the response options are ______

    A. Mutually exclusive
    B. Exhaustive

Questions 19–21

For each numbered study characteristic below, choose the most appropriate lettered answer. A given letter may be used once, more than once, or not at all.

Lettered response options: (Questions 19-21):

A. Cross-sectional study
B. Case-control study
C. Prospective cohort study
D. Historical cohort study

19. You would like to assess the effectiveness and efficiency of delivering health services through your clinic. After selecting a 10% sample of all patient visits during the past six months, you are able to characterize the patient population that is utilizing your clinic in terms of age, race, sex, method of referral, diagnostic category, therapy provided, method of payment, daily patient load, and clinic staff work schedules.

20. You are interested in finding out whether middle-aged men who have irregular heartbeats are at greater risk of developing a myocardial infarction (heart attack) than men whose heartbeats are regular. Electrocardiogram (ECG) examinations are subsequently performed on all male office employees 35 years of age or older who work for oil companies in Houston. The ECG tracings are classified as irregular or regular. Five years later, myocardial infarction rates are compared between those with and those without baseline ECG irregularities.

21. The entire population of a given community is examined, and all who are judged to be free from bowel cancer are questioned extensively about their diets. These people are then followed for several years to see whether or not their eating habits will predict their risk of developing bowel cancer.

Comprehensive Exam: Answers

1. D
2. A
3. A
4. A
5. A
6. A
7. A
8. C
9. C
10. D
11. C; case-control designs are the most efficient, since we "group" by disease status then "assess" exposure status
12. B; this question calls for "grouping" by exposure status then "assessing" disease status; given long-term effects and rare exposures, the retrospective cohort design is more efficient
13. C
14. A; this question calls for "grouping" by exposure status then "assessing" disease status; given a new exposure and short-term effects, the prospective cohort design is the better choice
15. C
16. A
17. B
18. A
19. A
20. C
21. C

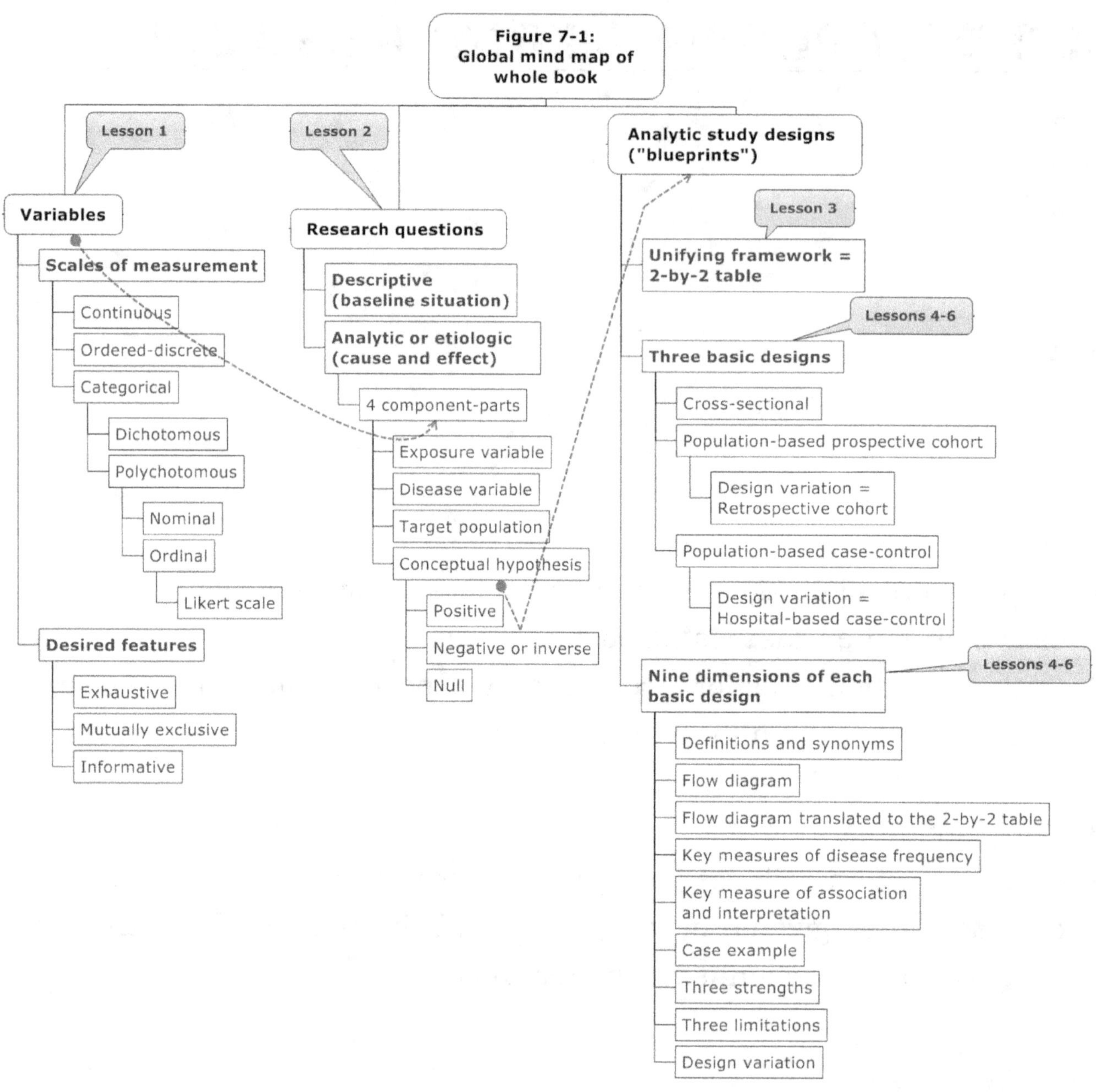
Figure 7-1:
Global mind map of
whole book
Lesson 1
Lesson 2
Variables
Scales of measurement
Continuous
Ordered-discrete
Categorical
Dichotomous
Polychotomous
Nominal
Ordinal
Likert scale
Desired features
Exhaustive
Mutually exclusive
Informative
Research questions
Descriptive
(baseline situation)
Analytic or etiologic
(cause and effect)
4 component-parts
Exposure variable
Disease variable
Target population
Conceptual hypothesis
Positive
Negative or inverse
Null
Analytic study designs
("blueprints")
Lesson 3
Unifying framework =
2-by-2 table
Lessons 4-6
Three basic designs
Cross-sectional
Population-based prospective cohort
Design variation =
Retrospective cohort
Population-based case-control
Design variation =
Hospital-based case-control
Lessons 4-6
Nine dimensions of each
basic design
Definitions and synonyms
Flow diagram
Flow diagram translated to the 2-by-2 table
Key measures of disease frequency
Key measure of association
and interpretation
Case example
Three strengths
Three limitations
Design variation

Worksheet 7-1: Alphabetical Lists of Terms

Instructions: Define each term below in your own words.

Lesson 1: Scales of Measurement

Categorical variable
Continuous variable
Dichotomous variable
Exhaustive
Informativeness
Likert scale
Mutually exclusive
Nominal variable
Ordered-discrete variable
Ordinal variable
Polychotomous variable
Variable

Lesson 2: From Variables to Research Questions

Analytic research question
Conceptual hypothesis
Dependent variable

Descriptive research question
Disease variable
Etiologic research question
Exposure variable
Independent variable
Inverse association
Negative association
Null association
Outcome variable
Positive association
Predictor variable
Research question
Response variable
Target population

Lesson 3: Analytic Study Designs and the 2-by-2 Table

Column marginal totals
Grand total
Row marginal totals
Standard 2-by-2 table
Study design

Lesson 4: The Cross-Sectional Study Design

Antecedent-consequence bias
Chicken-or-egg dilemma
Cross-sectional study design
Etiology
Incident cases
Point prevalence
Prevalence ratio (PR)
Prevalence study
Prevalent cases
Protective factor
Risk factor

Worksheet 7-1: Alphabetical Lists of Terms

Lesson 5: The Population-Based Prospective Cohort Study Design

Baseline
Confounding variables
Cumulative incidence
Follow-up study
Historical cohort design
Incidence study
Latency period
Longitudinal study
Losses to follow-up
Nonconcurrent cohort design
Population-based prospective cohort design
Population-based retrospective cohort design
Risk
Risk ratio (RR)

Lesson 6: The Population-Based Case-Control Design

Case-referent study
Catchment area
Exposure odds ratio (EOR)
Hospital-based case-control design
Odds
Population-based case-control design
Population-based disease registry
Recall bias
Surveillance Epidemiology and End Results (SEER) program

Bibliography

Abramson, J. H. *Making Sense of Data: A Self-Instruction Manual on the Interpretation of Epidemiologic Data.* New York: Oxford University Press, 1994.

Aday, L. A, and L. J. Cornelius. *Designing and Conducting Health Surveys: A Comprehensive Guide.* San Francisco: Jossey-Bass. 2006.

Ahlbom, A., and S. Norell. *Introduction to Modern Epidemiology.* Chestnut Hill: Epidemiology Resources Incorporated, 1984.

Aschengrau, A., and G. R. Seage. *Essentials of Epidemiology in Public Health.* Sudbury: Jones and Bartlett Publishers, 2008.

Booth, W. C., G. G. Colomb, and J. M. Williams. *The Craft of Research.* Chicago: The University of Chicago Press, 1995.

Friis, R. H., and T. A. Sellers. *Epidemiology for Public Health Practice.* Sudbury: Jones and Bartlett Publishers, 2009.

Gerstman, B. B. *Epidemiology Kept Simple: An Introduction to Traditional and Modern Epidemiology.* Hoboken: Wiley-Liss Incorporated, 2003.

Glaser, A. N. *High-yield Biostatistics.* Philadelphia: Lippincott Williams & Wilkins, 2005.

Gordis, L. *Epidemiology.* Philadelphia: Saunders Elsevier, 2009.

Greenberg, R. S., S. R. Daniels, W. D. Flanders, J. W. Eley, and J. R. Boring. *Medical Epidemiology.* New York: Lange Medical Books/McGraw-Hill, 2001.

Hennekens, C. H., and J. E. Boring. *Epidemiology in Medicine.* Boston: Little, Brown and Company, 1987.

Hulley, S. B., S. R. Cummings, W. S. Browner, D. G. Grady, and T. B. Newman. *Designing Clinical Research.* Philadelphia: Lippincott Williams & Wilkins, 2007.

Jekel, J. F., D. L. Katz, J. G. Elmore, and S. M. G. Wild. *Epidemiology, Biostatistics, and Preventive Medicine.* Philadelphia: Saunders Elsevier, 2007.

Katz, M. H. *Study Design and Statistical Analysis: A Practical Guide for Clinicians.* New York: Cambridge University Press, 2006.

Kirkwood, B. R., and J. A. C. Sterne. *Medical Statistics.* Malden (MA): Blackwell Science Ltd, 2003.

Kleinbaum, D. G., L. L. Kupper, and H. Morgenstern. *Epidemiologic Research: Principles and Quantitative Methods.* New York: Van Nostrand Reinhold Company, 1982.

Kleinbaum, D. G., K. M. Sullivan, and N. D. Baker. *ActivEpi Companion Textbook: A Supplement for Use with the ActivEpi CD-ROM.* New York: Springer, 2003.

——. *A Pocket Guide to Epidemiology.* New York: Springer, 2007.

Knapp, R. G., and M. C. Miller. *Clinical Epidemiology and Biostatistics.* Baltimore: Williams & Wilkins, 1992.

Kuzma, W., and S. E. Bohnenblust. *Basic Statistics for the Health Sciences.* New York: McGraw Hill, 2001.

Lang, T. A., and M. Secic. *How to Report Statistics in Medicine: Annotated Guidelines for Authors, Editors, and Reviewers.* Philadelphia: American College of Physicians, 2006

Last, J. M. *A Dictionary of Epidemiology.* New York: Oxford University Press, 1988.

Levine, D. M., and D. F. Stephan. *Even You Can Learn Statistics: A Guide for Everyone Who Has Ever Been Afraid of Statistics.* Upper Saddle River (NJ): Pearson Prentice Hall, 2005.

McDermott, R. J., and P. D. Sarvela. *Health Education Evaluation and Measurement: A Practitioner's Perspective.* New York: WCB/McGraw-Hill, 1999.

Novak, J. D., and D. B. Gowin. *Learning How to Learn.* New York: Cambridge University Press, 1994.

Ott, L., R. F. Larson, and W. Mendenhall. *Statistics: A Tool for the Social Sciences.* Boston: Duxbury Press, 1983.

Porta, M. *A Dictionary of Epidemiology.* New York: Oxford University Press, 2008.

Portney, L. G., and M. P. Watkins. *Foundations of Clinical Research: Applications to Practice.* Norwalk: Appleton & Lange, 1993.

Riegelman, R. K. *Studying a Study and Testing a Test: How to Read the Medical Evidence.* Philadelphia: Lippincott Williams & Wilkins, 2000.

Schlesselman, J. J. *Case-control Studies: Design, Conduct, Analysis.* New York: Oxford University Press, 1982.

Schulz, K. F., and D. A. Grimes. "Case-control Studies: Research in Reverse." The Lancet 359 (2002): 431–434.

Szklo, M., and F. J. Nieto. *Epidemiology Beyond the Basics.* Sudbury: Jones and Bartlett Publishers, 2007.

About the Author

Dr. Faulkner is a professor of epidemiologic science who is popular among her students, not only because of her passion for the field but also because of her down-to-earth techniques for making mathematics accessible to all.

www.ingramcontent.com/pod-product-compliance
Lightning Source LLC
Chambersburg PA
CBHW081240180526
45171CB00005B/489
* 9 7 8 1 4 7 9 3 6 9 5 5 3 *